LIPS

BY NATASHA DEVEDLAKA-PRICE

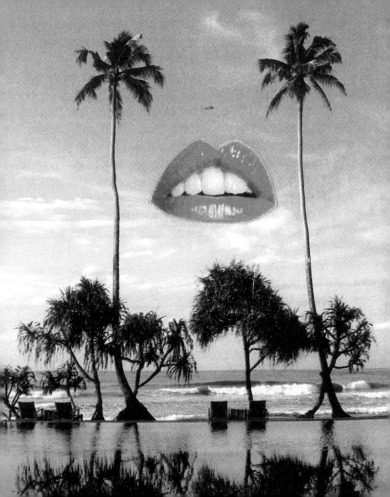

BY NATASHA DEVEDLAKA-PRICE

PHOTOGRAPHY BY MICK ACKLAND
AND CASEY MOORE

LIPS

HOW TO WEAR LIPSTICK, LIP GLOSS AND LIFT YOUR LIP GAME

hardie grant books

CONTENTS

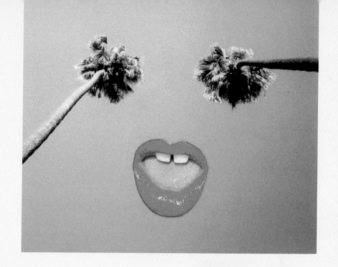

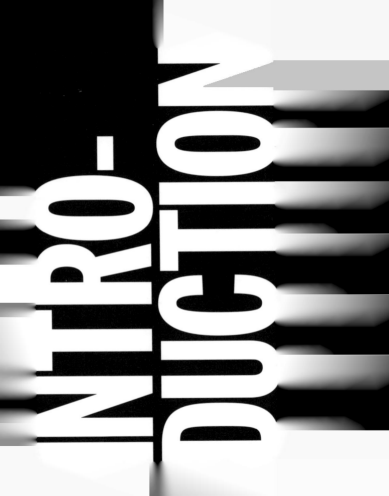

INTRO-
DUCTION

The mouth speaks volumes even without words – an awkward side smile, a pout – and simply adding a swipe of lipstick can boost your confidence, lift your mood and completely change your face.

My grandma was a 'put-on-your-lippy-to-greet-the-postman' kind of gal, and she's totally to blame for my unadulterated, joyful obsession. A Dior fuchsia pink was her favourite and she even wore it camping!

The adage of 'putting on your war paint' is so apt when it comes to lippy. Lipstick is your make-up armour – it has its own secret language and the power to transform any look with effortless impact. This book is a celebration of lipstick, and is filled with all sorts of tricks and tips to up your lip game. I hope you enjoy it!

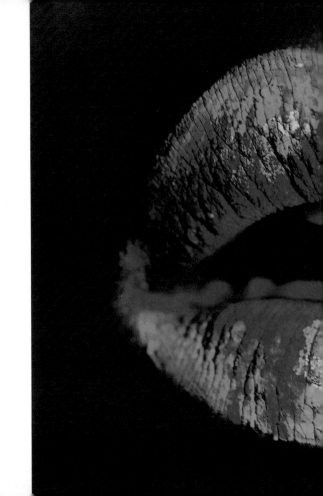

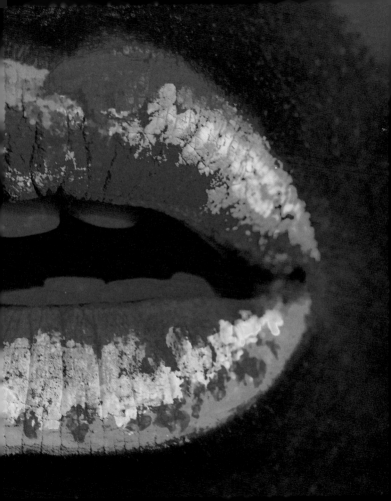

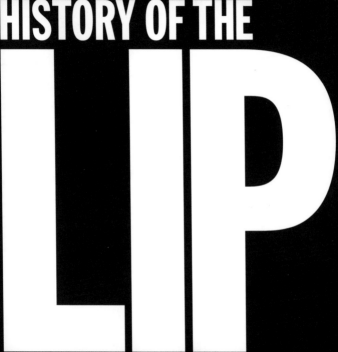

HISTORY OF THE
LIP

There's nothing new about lipstick – it's believed that Ancient Mesopotamian women were decorating their lips as far back as 2500 BC. Cleopatra famously painted her well-defined pout a bright red, using crushed insects mixed with beeswax. Post Ancient Egypt, lipstick went in and out of fashion until the 1900s, when it became an important part of women's daily attire.

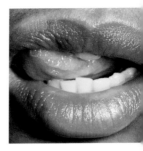

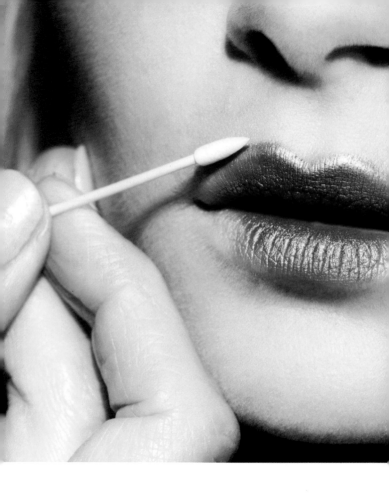

At first, the colouring of lips was discreet, but as women gained more social independence in the 1920s, the painting of lips went public. Inspired by the actress Clara Bow, lipstick became symbolic of the 'It' girl.

By the 1950s, chemist Hazel Bishop invented long-lasting, non-smearing, kiss-proof lipstick – immortalised in the line, 'It stays on you… not on him'. Film stars like Marilyn Monroe and Elizabeth Taylor only increased the popularity of lipstick, prompting cosmetics companies Max Factor and Revlon to create a whole new range of colours.

Today, L'Oréal and Estée Lauder dominate the lipstick market, while fashion houses like Chanel and YSL boast their own. Sales of lippy just keep booming, and there's even a theory that they increase during a recession. With all the colours of the rainbow, from gloss to matte, lipstick remains a fashion staple and a byword for femininity.

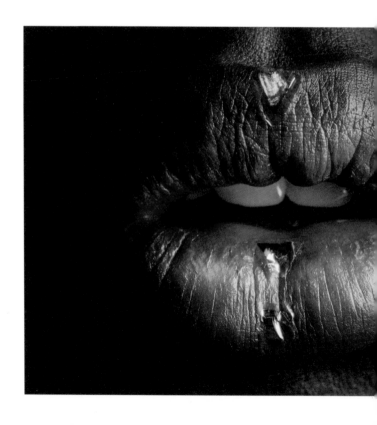

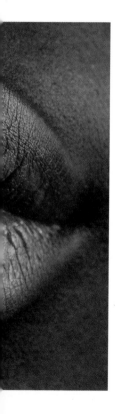

LIP PIERCING AND ADORNMENT

Today, lip piercings and adornments have become a common practice. They reflect a sense of individual style and personality.

Lip piercing originated from various African and South American tribes. Pierced adornments of the lip were sported by the Tlingit as well as people of Papua New Guinea and Amazonia. Aztecs and Mayans also wore labrets, while the Dogon people of Mali and the Nuba of Ethiopia wore rings.

Do your research before getting any piercings. Always go to a qualified piercer who uses a hollow needle and not a gun.

PART ONE

LIP CARE

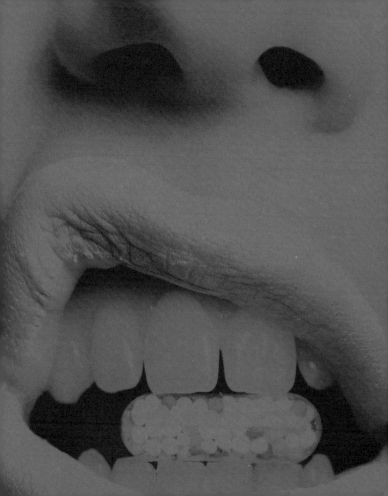

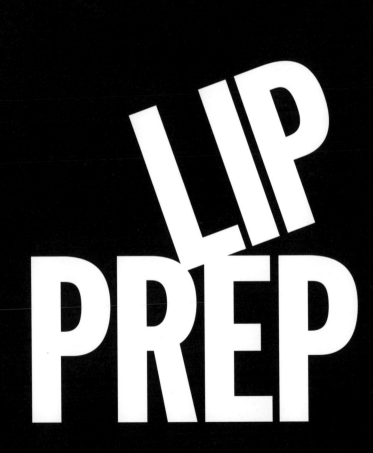

Taking good, general
care of your lips means
your mouth will always
be lipstick-ready.
For instance, a gentle
exfoliation can go a
long way to creating a
smooth and supple base
for your favourite lippy.
As well as this, your lips
may sometimes need a
little extra TLC if they've
been sunburnt or are
chapped. Follow the tips
on the following pages
to give your lips the best
care possible.

EXFOLIATE

Exfoliating your lips will ensure they won't chap. As lips are sensitive, do this once or twice a week. There are three easy ways to exfoliate your lips:

1. Use a natural, gentle scrub like Lush's Bubblegum Lip Scrub.

2. Buff a warm flannel over your lips.

3. Dip a children's toothbrush in coconut oil and brush it over your lips.

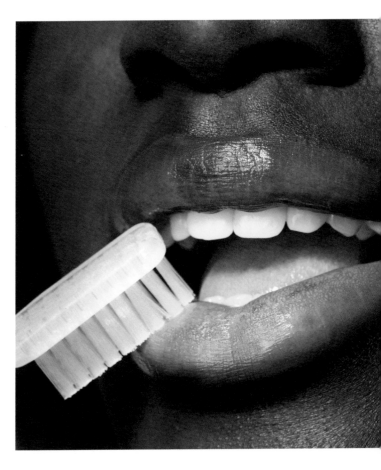

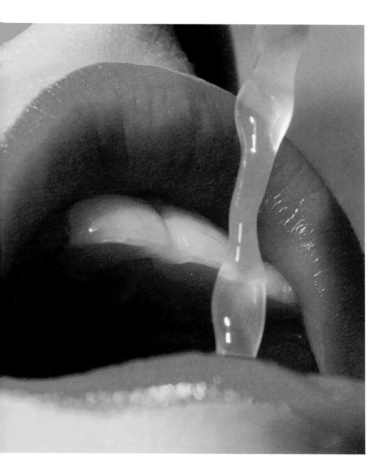

HYDRATE

Lipstick won't apply evenly to dry skin. Keeping lips hydrated will help to plump up your lips and keep them supple. To stay hydrated:

1. Drink plenty of water.

2. Use a humidifier in your bedroom at night to help keep your skin and lips hydrated and supple.

3. Don't lick your lips too much, as this makes them more vulnerable to the elements.

Lips lack natural protection

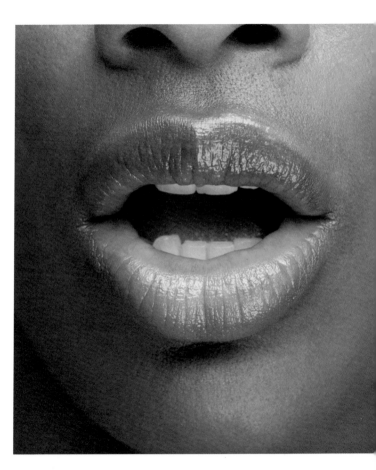

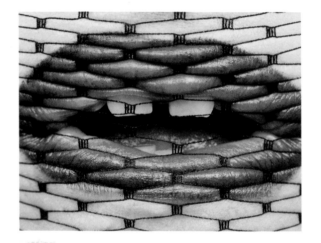

SUN PROTECTION

Always protect your lips from the sun – it's really damaging, and you run the risk of skin cancer:

1. Your lips have no melanin and will easily burn. Wear a hat and use a balm with a sun protection factor (SPF) of at least 30.

2. Too much sun will cause flaky, dry lips. It is best to cover your face with a cotton cloth when sunbathing and keep applying sunscreen, expecially if you're in water.

3. Overexposure to the sun (and smoking) can cause cat's arse mouth (wrinkles on the lips), which is extremely ageing!

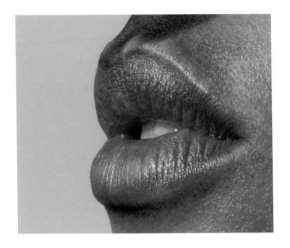

BALMS

Lip balm is an essential piece of make-up kit – it keeps lips supple – so invest in a good one.

Choose products that naturally hydrate, such as beeswax, coconut oil, clary balm, shea butter and olive oil.

Have rest days between lipsticks and keep long-stay lip products for occasional use only. If you have sensitive lips, stick to more natural lipsticks. There are lots of good ones out there. Try Burt's Bees lips in Napa Vineyard and Sedona Sands, and Lush lipstick in Ambition and Decisive.

WARNING: some lip balms can cause chapped lips. Avoid petroleum jelly, as it suffocates the skin, and mineral oil, which coats the skin with a plastic-like layer.

SPECIAL CARE

Sometimes your lips need some extra-special TLC:

Lips can crack, especially when exposed to excessive ultraviolet light, central heating, cold weather or wind. This makes them more vulnerable to infections and cold sores. If this happens to you, ditch the lipstick for a few days and gently exfoliate your lips (see page 20).

People with eczema and other allergies may find that their lips are more likely to crack in the corners. Dermatologists call this 'angular cheilitis' and it may need specialist treatment with an anti-inflammatory steroid or antibiotics if infection sets in. See your doctor if this occurs.

Don't forget that by drawing attention to your mouth, you are also drawing attention to your teeth. Ensure that you practise good dental care for a sparkling white smile.

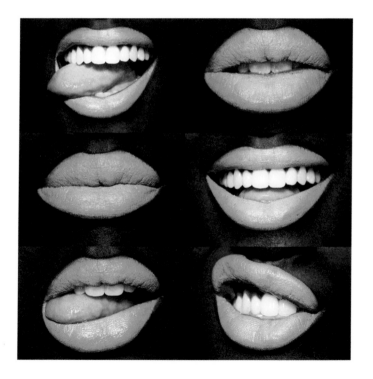

Lips project a lot of personality

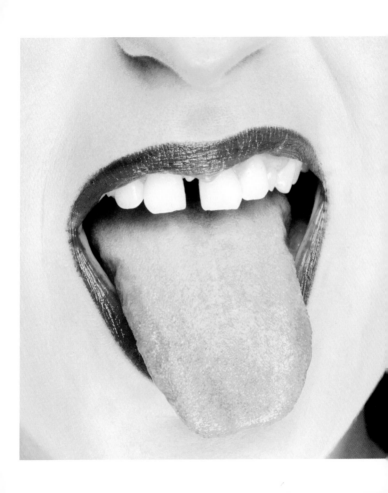

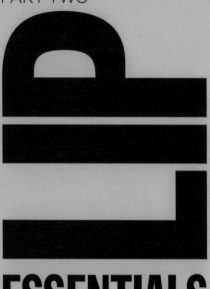

PART TWO

LIP

ESSENTIALS

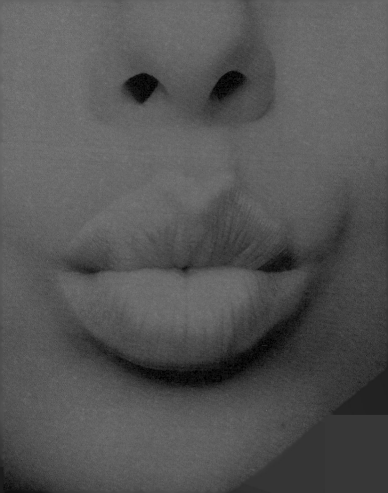

Your basic lip kit should include everyday items, no just for embellishment but also for care.

BASIC
KIT

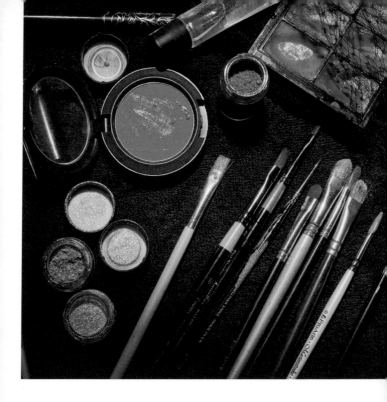

Lip balm – with SPF
Primer – to help your colour stay put
Liners – clear and pigmented
Lipsticks – matte and gloss,

cheap and expensive
Pigments and eye shadows – to add extra colour or shine
Brushes – flat, pointed,

oval (they don't have to be lip brushes)
Powder puff – to finish
Pointed cotton buds – to clean and tidy

THE
PERFECT
LIP

Lips come in all
different shapes
and sizes, but
if you apply your
lipstick correctly
it really can
make all the
difference. In
this section you
will learn how
to apply lip liner
and lipstick like
a pro, and even
change the shape
of your lips.

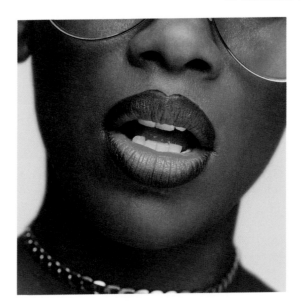

LIP LINER

What would Marilyn Monroe, Mae West, Pamela Anderson and the
Spice Girls have done without lip liner? Lip liner is the ultimate tool – it
can define, contour, shape and prevent colour from bleeding onto the face.
When used properly, lip liner is a must-have for your make-up kit,
and it's definitely lipstick's partner in crime.

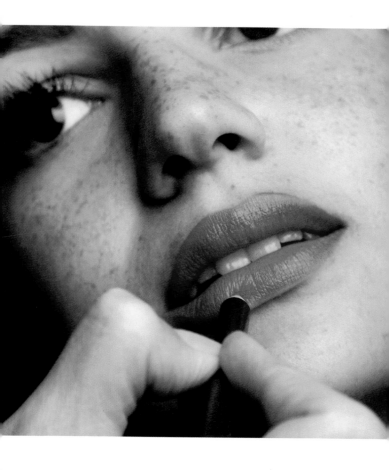

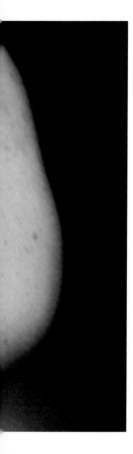

LIP LINER: SMART TIPS

TIP 1
Always match your lip liner to either your natural lip colour or your lipstick.

TIP 2
Use the tip of the lip pencil for your Cupid's bow and the edge of the tip for the rest of the mouth. Use the line of your mouth as a guide.

TIP 3
If you find lining your lips tricky, it can be easier to apply lip liner after lipstick.

TIP 4
Use your fingertip to blend the line for a more natural look.

TIP 5
Flesh-toned lip pencil applied all over the lips works well as 'no make-up' make-up.

TIP 6
Warm the tip of the pencil on the back of your hand for a more blendable line.

TIP 7
Lip pencil applied all over the lips makes a good base for balm and lip gloss.

TIP 8
Use it to highlight your lips' natural curve or change your lip shape (see page 50).

APPLYING LIPSTICK

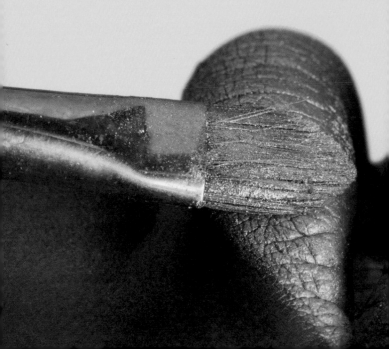

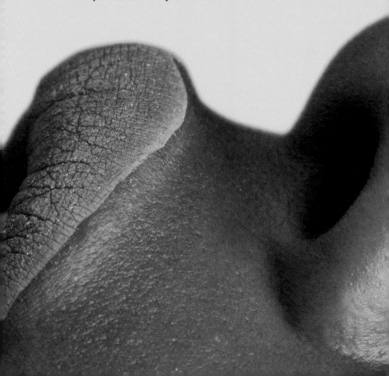

The first thing to do when applying lipstick or lip liner is to prep and prime your lips. Covering up chapped lips with lipstick will only accentuate the cracks.

To get a clean, polished look like the finish
in the photograph below, you need to follow
several crucial steps in lipstick application.
Once you get the hang of it, you'll be putting
on your pout in a flash!

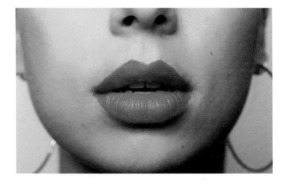

1. EXFOLIATE

Using lip balm has its benefits, but regular exfoliation removes any
dead skin, leaving that soft, plump finish. Just as with the rest of your
skin, moisturiser is great, but exfoliating is the real secret to soft,
smooth skin. See page 20 for my exfoliating tips – it's really quick
and easy to add to your beauty routine, I promise!

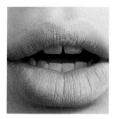

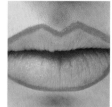

2. LIP PRIMER

3. LIP LINER

Once you have exfoliatied, you can further prep your lips with a lip primer, which will not only help the lipstick to glide on, but will ensure it stays put that little bit longer.

It's inevitable that your lipstick will fade slightly throughout the day or night, but a good primer will reduce this from happening.

MAC's Prep + Prime Lip not only extends the colour, but helps to smooth out lips and prevents it from bleeding (running outside of your lip line). Urban Decay's Lip Primer Potion is another great product.

Lip liner also increases the longevity of your lipstick, as well as adding definition and preventing bleeding. Try to find a lip liner that matches your choice of lipstick colour. Brands will have similar colours in both products for this exact reason.

Follow my tips on page 41 to learn how to line your lips like a pro.

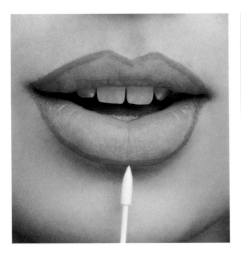

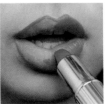

Directly applying lipstick from the tube is a quick method that results in a thick layer of pigment. It's fine to use this method with sheer and light textures. Pick a lipstick with a point or flat tip for more accuracy.

Lip brushes give you definition and precision, and I definitely recommend using one when applying strong colours and re-shaping your lips. It's also easier to apply lipstick to another person using a brush.

4. TIDY UP

If you have made any mistakes or want to clean up your lip line, you can take a concealer brush or cotton bud and apply a small amount of cream concealer, where needed. Blend it into the skin and your lips will pop!

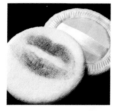

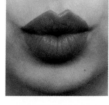

6. BLOT

7. GLOSS

There are ways to stop your lipstick from coming off or smudging after application. First, you can place your index finger in your mouth with your lips pressed down, then pull it out – this will stop lipstick from getting on your teeth. You can also take a single-ply tissue, place it gently over your lips, then with a large brush, dab on a small amount of loose translucent powder over the lips through the tissue. This works as a 'coating' for the lipstick. Lastly, you can take a tissue and bite your lips down on it for a couple of seconds.

For a moist, plump effect, add some gloss on top. Either add a gloss that's the same colour as your lipstick, of use a clear one. If you opt for clear, apply it with a lip brush so that your gloss doesn't get stained by the lipstick colour.

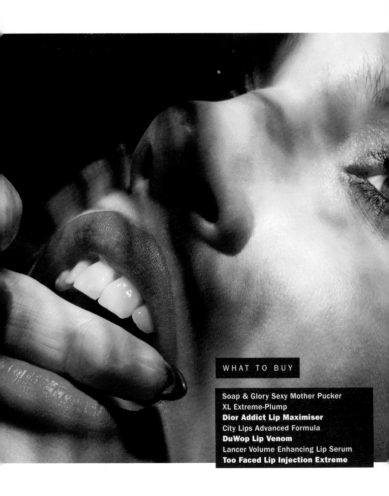

WHAT TO BUY

Soap & Glory Sexy Mother Pucker
XL Extreme-Plump
Dior Addict Lip Maximiser
City Lips Advanced Formula
DuWop Lip Venom
Lancer Volume Enhancing Lip Serum
Too Faced Lip Injection Extreme

CREATE A PLUMPER POUT

For fuller, plumper lips, follow the steps below:

1. Prep and prime lips (see pages 44–45).

2. Dab a little concealer on the lip line, blending it in lightly with your finger.

3. Lip liner is your friend! With caution, you can overline your lips slightly to create the illusion of a bigger pout.

4. Use either a soft satin or creamy finish lipstick.

5. Enjoy your enhanced pout!

CREATE A NEW SHAPE

Changing the shape of your lips is a really fun thing to try for a special occasion.

1. You'll need to make your lips a blank canvas, so start by prepping them (see tips 1 and 2 on pages 44 and 45).

2. Blot off any excess moisture with a tissue, and buff a small amount of foundation onto your lips with a brush.

3. Next, powder your lips with a powder puff, dusting off any excess with a large brush.

4. Once you've decided the shape you want to go for, start drawing your line with a sharp pencil. Re-sharpen during application if necessary.

5. Even when creating a new shape, use the natural lip as a guide to keep the shape even. If you're making your lips larger, stick to matte lipsticks to minimise the natural lip line.

6. If you're going for something dramatic, use tape as a stencil or your lip brush as a ruler to help get the shape you want.

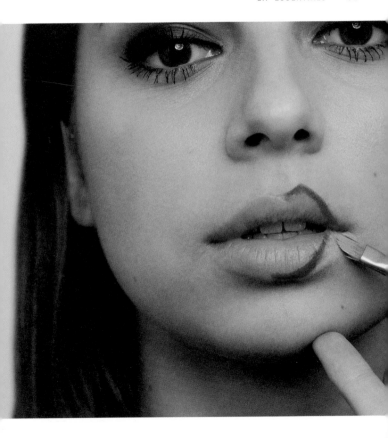

BUYING LIPSTICK

A good lipstick can brighten up your whole look. However, finding a shade that suits you can be a huge challenge. You may be surprised at how different colours actually look once applied to the lip – pigmentation varies amongst brands, so something that looks bright may not deliver. The best advice is to just take your time and try a few different brands and shades. Have fun with colour – you'll soon know if it's right by trusting your gut reaction when you see it on for the first time.

Things to keep in mind before making a purchase:

What's your first impression when
you see yourself?
Do your teeth look white or yellow?
Does your skin look fresh and your eyes bright?
Do you like the colour?
Does the texture feel good?

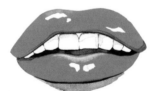

Thick vs thin lips:

Thinner lips can still wear reds; just stick to
brighter shades like cherry and orange reds.
If your lips are big, keep in mind that bright
shades will make them look larger.

DETERMINING SKIN TONE

Before you choose your lipstick colour, work out your skin tone.

Your skin tone can affect the way different lip shades play against your colouring. One quick way to determine your skin's undertone is by peeking at the inside of your wrist to see if you have blue or green veins. Blue indicates cool undertones, while green indicates warm. If you're still not sure, do a quick Google search of the foundation you use, and that should help you out.

People with cool undertones should try brighter reds with a bluish cast, and those with warm undertones should experiment with oranges and corals.

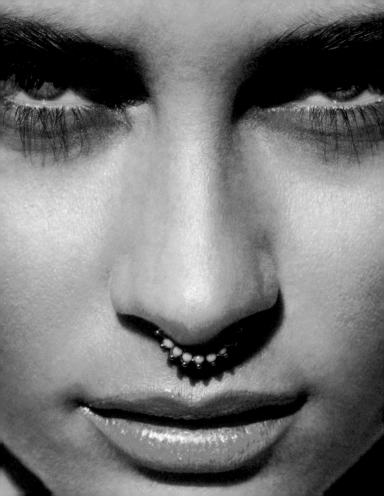

CHOOSING THE

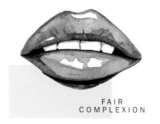

FAIR
COMPLEXION

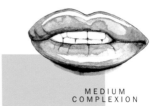

MEDIUM
COMPLEXION

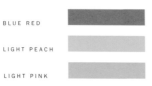

BLUE RED

LIGHT PEACH

LIGHT PINK

BLOOD RED

PEACH

PINK

RIGHT COLOUR

The best advice I can give is that you should play around with colour, but here are the basics on what will suit your skin tone.

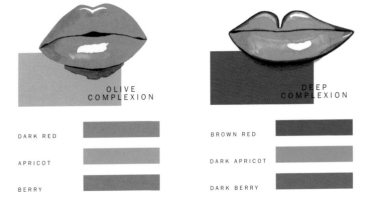

OLIVE
COMPLEXION

DARK RED

APRICOT

BERRY

DEEP
COMPLEXION

BROWN RED

DARK APRICOT

DARK BERRY

Lips are the most exposed erogenous zone!

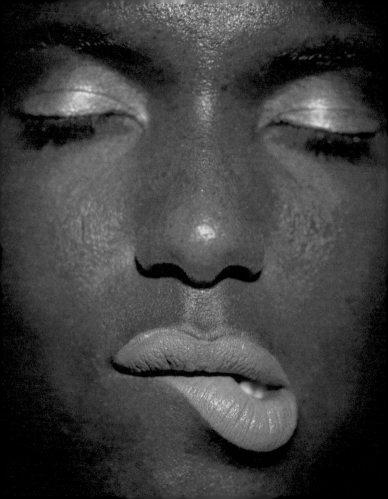

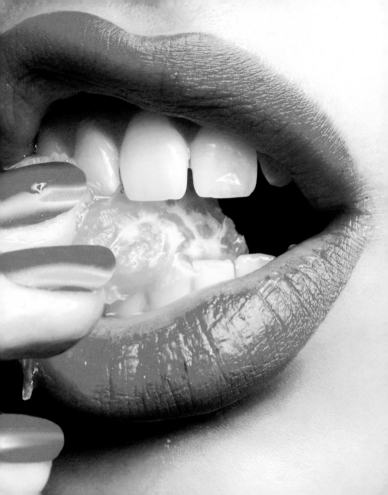

TRICKS OF THE LIGHT

Light reflects off creamy and glossy textures, giving the illusion of volume. Keep this in mind when painting your lips, to get the maximum pout effect.

Shades that match your skin tone are best to create the impression of fullness, and also look the most natural.

Generally speaking, the glossier the lipstick, the less time it will stay on your mouth, so be prepared to reapply. Matte lipsticks can make lips look and feel thinner, as they lack oils and are a lot drier than glossier, creamier lipsticks.

If you are drawing over your lip line, matte lipstick will disguise this better – just keep it a light shade.

Investing in a good, clear lip gloss can double your lipstick wardrobe.

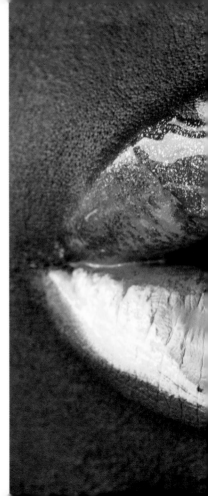

TEXTURES

Matte
Highly pigmented. Gives no shine at all and is long-lasting. It also comes in liquid form, which is easier to apply and not as drying.

Gloss
High-shine, glassy and sticky. Gives an instant look of fullness. Not long-lasting.

Satin/Sheer
Light coverage, colour and texture. These lipsticks need constant touch-ups but are really moisturising.

Frost/Shimmer
Highly pigmented, with shine and light reflectivity. Moisturising, medium-wear.

Creamy
Great colour pay-off and really moisturising. Medium-wear.

Liquid Crème
Matte, highly pigmented and often waterproof; doesn't budge but can be drying.

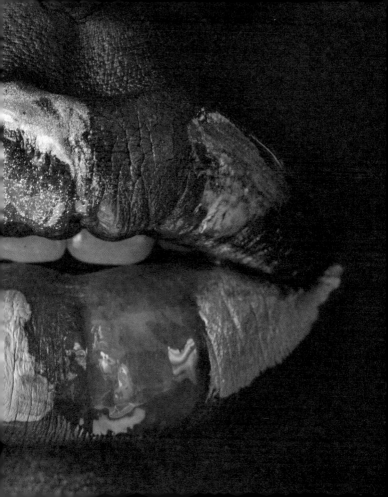

BARGAIN VS EXPENSIVE

Lipsticks can vary dramatically in price, so is it worth splurging or do the cheap brands do the job just as well?

It may seem that you are forking out for just the brand, but expensive lipsticks do often contain superior ingredients. Not only are they made with better moisturisers, such as shea butter and aloe vera extract, they may also have better pigmentation, staying ability and plumping power. Poor-quality pigment could make your lips look grey. Stronger pigmentation means your lipstick won't need to be reapplied as often, and will also have a bolder colour that will pop.

These days, cheaper brands are pretty good, but they also differ in smell and packaging and can stain your lips.

My advice is that if you're dipping into a trend, try out a cheaper brand. But if you're after a signature colour, go for the splurge.

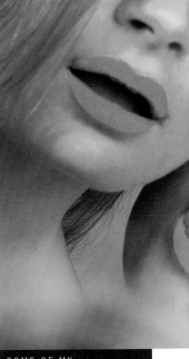

SOME OF MY
FAVOURITE BRANDS:

BARGAIN: Rimmel, NYX, Barry M

SPLURGE: YSL, Tom Ford, Chantecaille

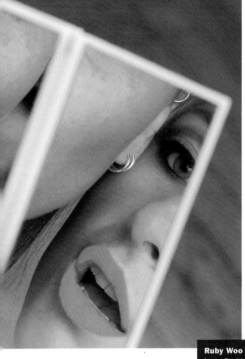

LIPSTICKS THAT SUIT ALL SKIN TONES

These Holy Grail lip shades suit everyone.

Ruby Woo by MAC – matte retro red
Iman Red by IMAN – semi-matte moisturising red
Dressed To Kill by NARS – fuschia rose with a gold shimmer
C-Thru Lipglass by MAC – clear lip gloss
Girl About Town by MAC – matte bright fuschia pink

As the skin ages it loses both hydration and collagen, so you need a little more care when it comes to prepping for and applying lipstick. Texture is important for more mature lips, so go for creamy, moisturising lipsticks. Glossy textures will inevitably bleed into those tiny creases that tend to form around more mature lips. Careful prep and using a lip liner, in particular, will pay dividends.

THE MATURE LIP

Prep and Conceal

Use a highlighting concealer along
the edges of lips to fill lines and
prevent feathering. YSL's Touche Éclat
does the trick.

Shape

It can feel like your lips are
disappearing as you get older. A lip
liner (see page 39) will help bring
them back to life. STUDIO 10 Age
Reverse Perfecting Lip Liner
is excellent.

Colours

Embrace colour! It immediately warms
and lifts the complexion. Dark shades
tend to make lips look thin, and pale
shades can make you look washed out,
so aim for something in between.

'I think getting old is a privilege. When I go to make-up counters they often say don't wear bright red lipstick at my age. I've never listened! It brightens up my face and outfit, and makes me feel cheerful.'

SUSAN **WILSON**

— ARTIST

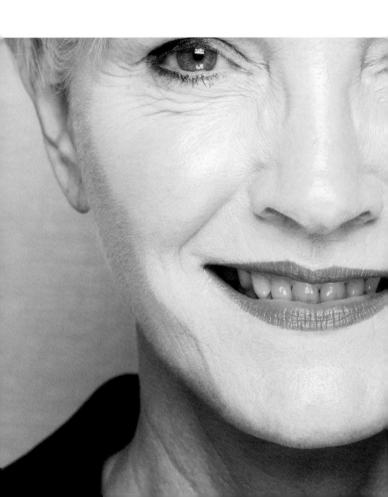

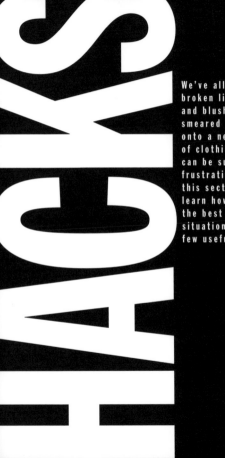

We've all broken lipsticks and blushes or smeared lippy onto a new item of clothing, which can be supremely frustrating. In this section, learn how to make the best of a bad situation with a few useful hacks.

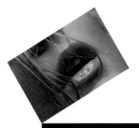

FIX A BROKEN LIPPY

If it's pretty new and in overall good condition:

1. Lay some paper towels down and pop on a pair of rubber gloves.

2. Gently remove the lipstick from the base.

3. Twist the lipstick up as far as possible, and heat the base using a match or lighter, being careful not to melt the case. Next, heat the broken end of the lipstick.

4. Once the lipstick has slightly melted, carefully place the broken lipstick back into the base.

5. Use a toothpick or match to blend the two parts together.

6. Chill in the fridge for 30 minutes, then use!

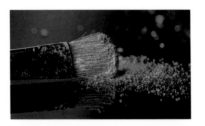

There's nothing worse than forking out on a new blush, only to drop it on the bathroom floor and smash it. Save the pieces and turn it into a new lip colour:

1. Pick up any salvageable pieces from the floor. Try not to cry.

2. Crush the pieces into a fine powder.

3. Add 1 teaspoon beeswax pastilles, 1 teaspoon shea or cocoa butter and 1 teaspoon coconut oil to a small glass bowl. Melt over a pan of simmering water until it becomes liquid. Mix in the crushed blush, adding more blush for a more intense colour.

4. Transfer the mixture to a small pot or jar. Allow to cool for 30 minutes before using.

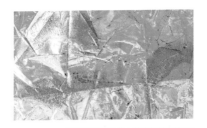

REMOVE A LIPPY STAIN

We've all done it: taken off a new shirt and rubbed it on our bright lips, causing a stain. Don't panic! It will come out if you follow the steps below:

1. Move quickly. Take off the item of clothing and check the care label. If it's washable, spray the stain generously with hairspray.

2. Let the hairspray sit on the stain for around 15 minutes so it can break down the grease from the lipstick.

3. Take a clean cloth and dampen it with warm water. Dab the stain with the cloth to loosen the colour from the fabric. You should see it disappearing.

4. Wash as usual.

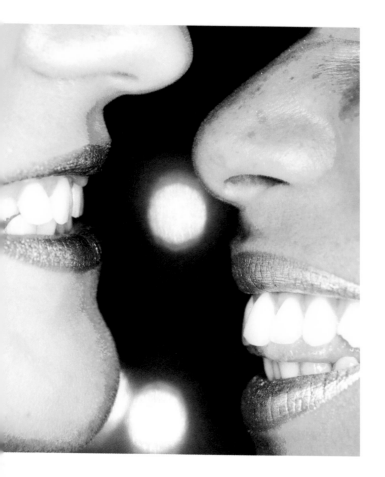

Kissing releases endorphins, which creates a sense of euphoria

PART THREE

THE COLOURS

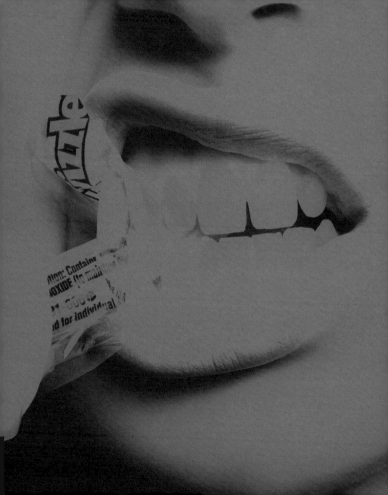

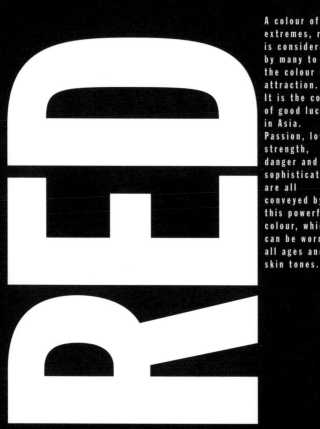

RED

A colour of extremes, red is considered by many to be the colour of attraction. It is the colour of good luck in Asia. Passion, love, strength, danger and sophistication are all conveyed by this powerful colour, which can be worn by all ages and skin tones.

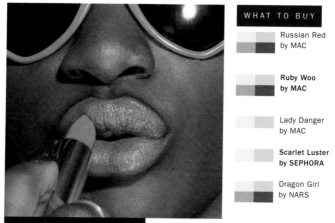

WHAT TO BUY

Russian Red
by MAC

**Ruby Woo
by MAC**

Lady Danger
by MAC

**Scarlet Luster
by SEPHORA**

Dragon Girl
by NARS

RED LIPS: SMART TIPS

TIP 1

Wear red lips
with minimal eye
make-up and
well-groomed
eyebrows.

TIP 2

Blue-toned reds
tend to make your
teeth look whiter.

TIP 3

For a sheer look,
dab red lipstick
onto your lips
using your finger.

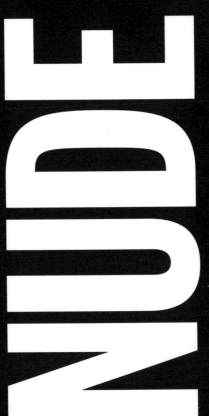

NUDE

These flesh-toned lipsticks resemble the colour of skin and are super sexy. Perfect for any aspiring Kylie Jenner or for a touch of understated 60s glamour.

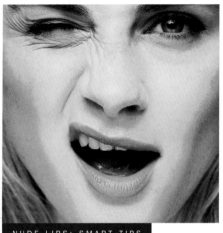

NUDE LIPS: SMART TIPS

WHAT TO BUY

Kinda Sexy by MAC

Rosepout
by Illamasqua

K.I.S.S.I.N.G Stoned Rose by Charlotte Tilbury

Lasting Finish
by Kate, Nude #44,
by Rimmel

**Nude Kate
by Charlotte Tilbury**

Rouge in Love in
Cocoa Couture by
Lancôme

Fresh Brew by Mac

TIP 1

To ensure natural
nude lipstick, dab
a small amount
of foundation
over the top with
your finger.

TIP 2

If your nude lippy
is washing you
out, add gloss
and extra blush
to your cheeks to
revive it.

TIP 3

Go for a couple of
shades darker for
a natural polished
look, or a couple
of shades lighter
for a sexier look.

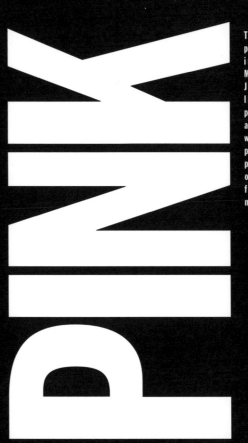

PINK

The colour pink is loved in India, Morocco and Japan. Pink lips can be playful, sweet and fresh. Try wearing pale pink for a pretty look, or a hot pink for something more vibrant.

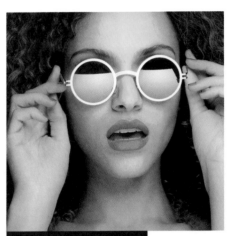

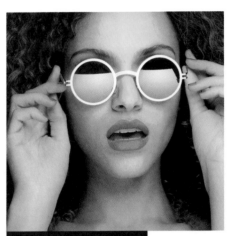

WHAT TO BUY

Hug Me by MAC

Saint Lipstick Hot Rose by Lipstick Queen

Show Orchid by MAC

Bright Rose by Lancôme

PINK LIPS: SMART TIPS

TIP 1

If wearing a hot pink, use minimal or no blush in order to avoid overloading the face.

TIP 2

If wearing a pale pink, you'll need to add warmth to your face. Try adding a coral blush or bronzer.

TIP 3

Check whether the colour works for you, as pale pink can make teeth look yellow.

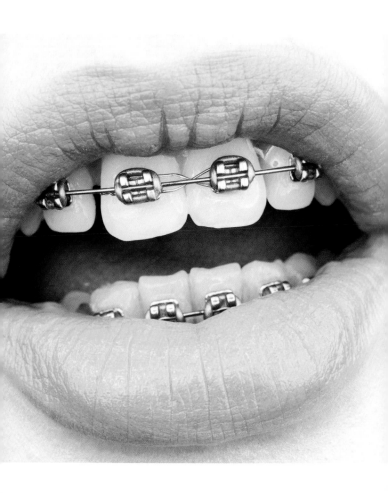

Lips are one of the most sensitive parts of the body

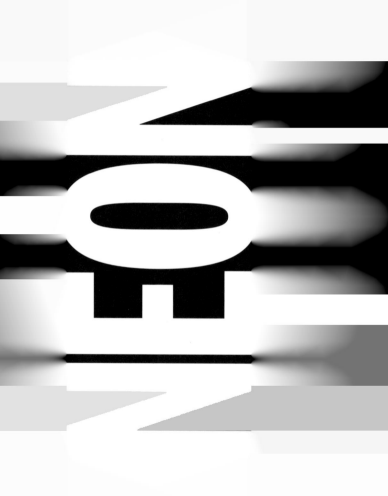

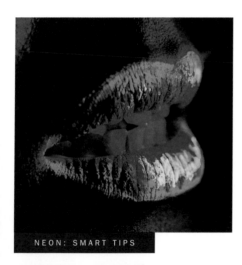

NEON: SMART TIPS

Neon paints from brands such as Fardel and Kryolan will glow under black light and can be used in place of make-up as they're non-toxic. You can use a UV torch to check their intensity.

If you don't want to go full-on neon, try lipsticks near to neon. MAC has two lip shades I recommend: Neon Orange and Candy Yum-Yum.

You can also try patting some pure pigments over your base lipstick with your finger. MAC's Genuine Orange or Process Magenta are great.

TIP 1

Neon paints dry quickly, so you'll need to work fast.

TIP 2

Neon lips are like camo – they suit every skin tone!

TIP 3

Paint lips before the rest of your make-up, as the slightest speck of neon will show up under UV light.

ORANGE

The colour of adventure, orange lips are bright and bold. The perfect colour to keep the summer blues at bay, a pop of orange lippy adds warmth to every skin tone, and can be worn all year round.

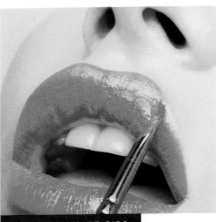

ORANGE: SMART TIPS

WHAT TO BUY

K.I.S.S.I.N.G.
Coachella Coral by
Charlotte Tilbury

Morange by
MAC

#23 Coral
Poetique by YSL

#29 Latin Lover
by SEPHORA

Timanfaya by
NARS

TIP 1

If you're buying
orange lipstick for
the first time, dip
in with a sweet
coral, which suits
most skin tones.

TIP 2

It's best to keep
the rest of your
make-up simple
when wearing a
bold orange.

TIP 3

The key to
mastering orange
lips is precise
application:
invest in a clear
or orange lip liner.

BLACK

Black lips are secretive, mysterious, Goth, spacey, strong, powerful, elegant and forever cool.

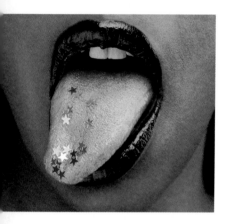

WHAT TO BUY

Cyber Dark Purple
by MAC

Kale by Bite Beauty

Witches by Kat
Von D

Black Velvet Matte
Velvetine by Lime
Crime

TIP 1

Black lips will
transform any
look. Just try it,
you may feel like
a badass!

TIP 2

It's easier to
apply black
lipstick first, then
lip liner.

TIP 3

Lip liner is
definitely needed
for black lips (you
can use a black
eyeliner).

TIP 4

You may need two
to three coats
to get an even
colour.

TIP 5

Smile and reapply
lipstick to fill any
creases.

TIP 6

If adding gloss,
dab it on, as
rubbing can
cause colour to
shift, resulting in
streaking.

TIP 7

If you feel black
is too much for
your complexion,
opt for an almost-
black, such as
very dark purple.

TIP 8

Always add a
warm blush or
bronzer to your
face if opting for
dark lips, to give
your face colour.

BURGUNDY

With red wine, dark purple and chocolate undertones, burgundy is the ultimate in grown-up glamour — warm and classy.

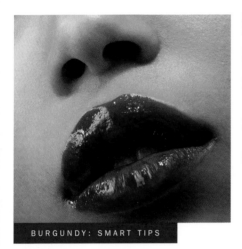

BURGUNDY: SMART TIPS

WHAT TO BUY

Glastonberry by Charlotte Tilbury

Lasting Finish by Kate shade 09 by Rimmel

Damned by Kat Von D

Vamp by MDMflow

TIP 1

Darker lipsticks usually need two coats to achieve an even finish.

TIP 2

Keep your make-up simple, but don't skimp on blusher as dark lips can wash you out.

TIP 3

Burgundy lipsticks have different undertones: purple, brown and red.

Your lips are unique to you, just like your fingerprints

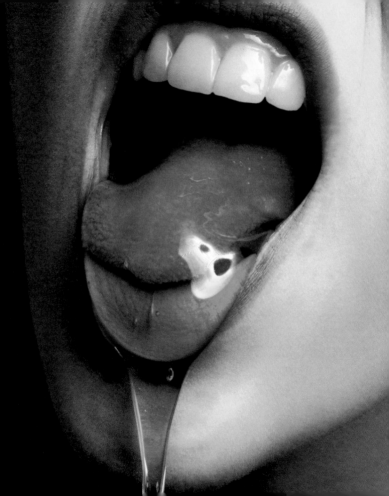

METALLIC

Futuristic
cyber-goth:
it's time to
be daring and
embrace this
fun lip trend.

TIP 1

Metallic lipstick looks amazing in daylight, so it's perfect for festivals.

TIP 2

Dab a non-toxic metallic eye shadow over a lipstick you already own to add a hint of shine. Make sure it is safe to use on your lips!

TIP 3

Metallic eyeliners also double up as lip liners. Urban Decay's 24/7 Glide-On eye pencils are excellent for this.

TIP 4

Balance is the key. The more metallic your lips, the less flashy the rest of your make-up should be. Matte skin complements metallic lips.

TIP 5

For the full metallic look, try NYX Cosmic Metals or Mehron Metallic Powder. If you don't want to go full metallic, try a gloss with just a hint of shine. YSL Gloss Volupte in Gold or Maybelline's Color Sensational Lip range are both great.

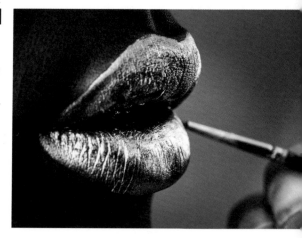

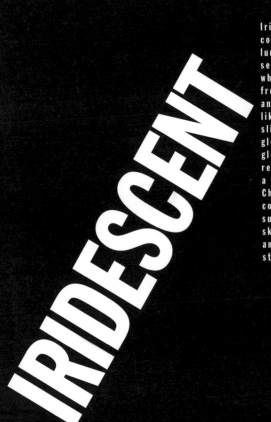

IRIDESCENT

Iridescent colours are luminous, and seem to change when seen from different angles, almost like an oil slick. Shining, gleaming and glowing, they really make a huge impact. Choose a base colour that suits your skin tone, and follow the steps opposite.

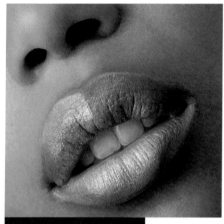

IRIDESCENT TIPS

WHAT TO BUY

For just a hint of iridesence, non-toxic, lip-safe metallic eye shadows and pigment are great for all skin tones. Try:

Holographic Stick by Milk Makeup

Firebird (Cream) by Urban Decay

TIP 1

The best iridescent lips can be achieved by mixing your own colours. Experiment with some non-toxic, lip-safe metallic eye shadows.

TIP 2

Pick a matte lip colour for your base. Then apply one or two lighter shades as you work towards the centre of your lips, blending with a brush.

TIP 3

The final step is what adds the magic: the top glossy coat. Gently apply a high-shine lip gloss for the full oil-slick mermaid lip effect.

You probably already own the tools to achieve this look: all you need are two lipsticks of a similar shade, one noticeably darker than the other. The colour gradually becomes lighter or darker towards the edges of your lips, resulting in a strong highlight. Go as natural or as bold as you fancy.

OMBRÉ/
FADE

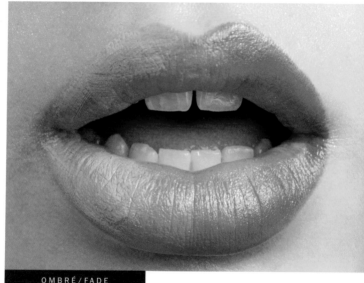

OMBRÉ/FADE

TIP 1

The most wearable and flattering ombré is dark around the edges, fading to light. Line your lips with the darker colour to begin.

TIP 2

Apply the darker base coat of lipstick. Next, add the lighter colour to the centre of your lips, gradually applying less pigment as you move outwards.

TIP 3

Press your lips together to further blend the lipsticks together. Check in the mirror and touch up any visible gaps of colour.

Think beyond the beauty hall and look to craft and haberdashery shops for materials and art books for inspiration. Experiment with tools, colours and textures to get different effects.

LIP PLAY

EASY LIP PATTERN

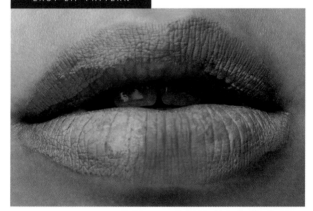

TIP 1

For best results, try using two bold colours on a matte lipstick base. Pigments are great to pat on top.

TIP 2

If you're not crazy about the pattern you've created, rub your lips together for a whole new colour and design.

TIP 3

Try using lace, net and stencils to create patterns. Use tape and tiny cotton buds to clean and correct any mistakes.

TIP 4

It's not all about being neat and tidy – going outside your lip line can add to your unique, one-off look.

Glitter is
not just for
Christmas!
Sparkly lips
grab attention
all year round.

GLITTER

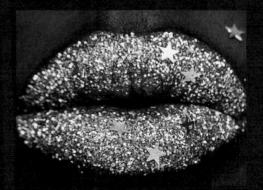

APPLICATION

1. Prep and prime your lips (see pages 44–45).

2. Apply lipstick (not gloss, otherwise the glitter will slide) and lip liner.

3. Choose your glitter. Ensure that you always use glitter that is specially formatted for use on the face. Mix different sized pieces and colours of glitter for a more theatrical look, or use one type of glitter for a showgirl look.

4. Dip an eye shadow sponge applicator in water so it is damp but not dripping.

5. If working on another person, ask them to lie down for easier application. Press the damp applicator into the glitter and pat it onto the lips. Use tape to remove any excess glitter from the face, and a cotton bud dipped in make-up remover to neaten up the lip line.

Once upon a time, there were certain colour combinations that were considered beauty no-nos. Thank goodness that's all changed!

PURPLE AND YELLOW

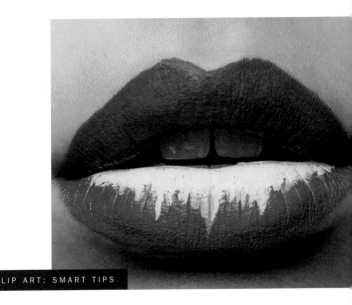

LIP ART: SMART TIPS

TIP 1

Start by applying the lighter colour with a brush. Clean the brush before applying the darker colour.

TIP 2

Remember not to press your lips together! And take your colours with you for touch-ups.

TIP 3

I also love silver with gold, black with navy, teal with fuchsia, and lilac with lime green.

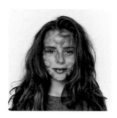

MASSIVE THANKS TO

My wonderful family! To my husband, Michael, for supporting me and producing the beautiful images for the book. To my son, George, for his practical brains and great chats. To Theodora, who is beautiful inside and out: thank you for being so wonderful!

Thanks to Kate Pollard at Hardie Grant for making it happen and supporting my ideas, and to Mary Lees for the stylish design. Sharmadean Reid, thanks for all the inspirational chats about everything under the sun. Thanks also to fellow lipstick-addict Sian Singer.

Thanks to Frances and Sam at Mac Pro, Carnaby Street. Thanks also to Tilde, Jo and Em for the hours of make-up I put you through as kids. And, finally, thanks go to Darren Evans for letting me assist you on my first make-up job.

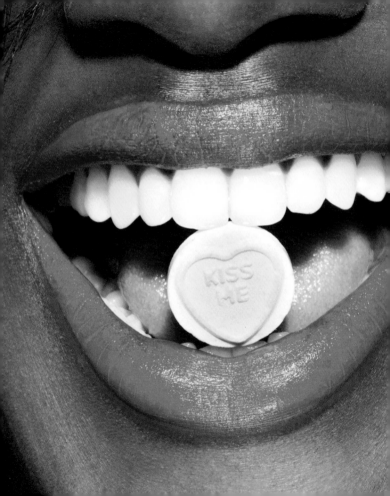

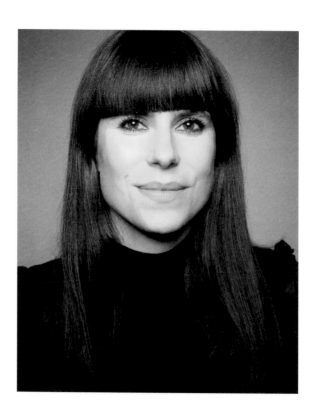

NATASHA DEVEDLAKA-PRICE

As a child, Natasha rubbed cherry brandy lollies onto her lips to stain them red. She's since moved on to actual lipsticks and hasn't looked back!

Natasha has been a make-up artist for over 20 years and has worked with people from Lily Allen to Barack Obama. She lives in London with her husband and two children.

@unruly_beauty_

Lips by Natasha Devedlaka-Price

First published in 2017 by Hardie Grant Books

Hardie Grant Books (UK)
52-54 Southwark Street
London SE1 1UN
hardiegrant.co.uk

Hardie Grant Books (Australia)
Ground Floor, Building 1
658 Church Street
Melbourne, VIC 3121
hardiegrant.com.au

British Library Cataloguing-in-Publication Data. A catalogue record for this book is available from
the British Library.

ISBN: 978-1-78488-101-6

Publisher: Kate Pollard
Senior Editor: Kajal Mistry
Editorial Assistant: Hannah Roberts
Publishing Assistant: Eila Purvis
Art Direction: Mary Lees
Photographers: Mick Ackland and Casey Moore
Nails: Keziah Waudby @wahnails
Models: Alexis, Barbra, Emily, Jennifer, Maddie, Polly, Sharea, Sharmadean, Stephanie, Tytiah,
Velenzia, Vicky, Zaneta
Colour Reproduction by p2d

Printed and bound in China by 1010

10 9 8 7 6 5 4 3 2 1